EAT
TO BEAT
DISEASE

Cookbook

Delicious and Easy-to-Make Recipes to Help Transform Your Health.

By

Lizzy j. Brown

Disclaimer:

The information provided in this book is designed to provide helpful information on the subjects discussed. The publisher and author are not responsible for any specific health or allergy needs that may require medical supervision and are not liable for any damages or negative consequences from any treatment, action, application or preparation, to any person reading or following the information in this book.

Table of Contents

INTRODUCTION:

The New Science of How Your Body Can Heal Itself

Nevertheless, we are truly at a turning point in the fight against disease. Each of us has the ability to take charge of our lives using food to transform our health. It is time to make decisions about what to eat and drink based on scientific evidence gleaned from testing foods with the same systems and methods that have been used to discover and develop drugs. Food can influence our health in specific and beneficial ways.

However, drug treatments alone cannot keep us healthy. Food is a better answer to preventing disease, before we have to cure it. Every doctor knows that unhealthy diet is linked to preventable disease, and food is becoming a topic of ever greater importance in the medical community.

What I clearly know is that our health is an active state, protected by a series of remarkable defense systems in the body that are firing on all cylinders, from birth to our last day alive, keeping our body cells and organs functioning perfectly. Remember that these health defense systems are hardwired in our body to protect us. While some are so powerful, they can even reverse diseases like cancer. And as they function as separate systems of defense, they also support and interact with one another. They are known to be the common denominators of health. So, by recalibrating our approach to preventing disease and focusing on these common denominators, we can take a unified approach to intercepting diseases before they set in.

Although you might have the knowledge that eating certain foods can increase your ability to beat disease. The eat to beat disease cookbook will be your perfect guide, whether you have years of unhealthy eating under your belt or you simply want to fine-tune your diet. Having the knowledge of which foods to eat more often and which foods to limit, you'll be on your way toward a healthy you.

THE EAT TO BEAT DISEASE RECIPES TO TRANFORM YOU

Delectable recipes for your Breakfast

Apple & cinnamon crepes served with Greek yoghurt

Ingredients

Apple filling:

1 tablespoon of water

2 ½ medium Granny Smith apples (peeled, cored and diced)

1 teaspoon of cinnamon

Crepes:

½ cup of reduced fat milk

1 tablespoon of honey

1 tablespoon honey (to serve)

1 egg

¾ cup of whole meal plain flour

Spray olive oil

4 tablespoons of reduced fat Greek yoghurt (to serve)

Directions:

Directions for Apple Filling:

1. First, place cinnamon, apples, and water in a medium sized saucepan over medium-low heat.
2. After which you bring to the boil; reduce heat to low.
3. After that, simmer, covered, for about 8-10 minutes or until apple is tender; set aside.

4. Then, in a large mixing bowl, whisk eggs, plain flour, milk, and honey and until mixture is smooth and lump free.
5. At this point, spray a large non-stick frying pan with olive oil and set over medium-high heat.
6. Furthermore, using a ladle, scoop approximately ½ cup batter into the pan and distribute the batter around the pan so the crepe is as thin as possible.
7. In addition, after 1-2 minutes or when little air bubbles appear, flip the crepe over using a spatula.
8. After that, cook on the other side for about 1-2 minutes and transfer to a plate.
9. Make sure you repeat for the remaining mixture.
10. Finally, if you want to serve, place crepe on a plate, top with apples and 1 tablespoon Greek yoghurt and a drizzle of honey.

Baked eggs with grainy toast

Ingredients

1 brown onion (finely chopped)

2 medium red capsicums (halved, seeded, thinly sliced length-ways)

1 tablespoon of ground coriander

4 ripe tomatoes (finely diced)

2 cups of baby spinach leaves

4 thick slices multigrain bread (to serve)

Spray olive oil

4 cloves garlic (peeled, sliced)

1 tablespoon of ground cumin

2 teaspoons of paprika

300g can no added salt kidney beans (drained, rinsed)

4 eggs

2 tablespoons of parsley (to serve)

Directions:

1. Meanwhile, heat oven to 180°C.
2. After which you spray a large non-stick frying pan with olive oil and set over medium-high heat.
3. After that, add onion and garlic to the pan cook for about 1-2 minutes, or until just softened.
4. Then, add cumin, capsicum, coriander and paprika and cook, stirring, for 2 minutes.
5. At this point, you add kidney beans, tomato and spinach and cook for 5 minutes.

6. Furthermore, divide capsicum, tomato and kidney bean mixture between 4 large ramekins.
7. This is when you use a spoon to create a well in the center of each ramekin.
8. In addition, crack 1 egg into each well.
9. After which you bake for about 10 minutes or until egg white is set and yolk remains soft.
10. Finally, you sprinkle with parsley and serve with grainy toast.

Tip:

Remember, the capsicum, tomato and kidney bean mix can be made ahead of time and reheated in the morning before adding the egg.

Banana French Toast

Ingredients

2 eggs

½ tablespoon of honey

Spray olive oil

1 tablespoon of sultanas

300g reduced fat Greek Yoghurt (to serve)

4 slices of whole meal bread

½ cup of reduced fat milk

½ teaspoon of vanilla extract

1 banana (sliced)

½ teaspoon of cinnamon

Directions:

1. Meanwhile, heat oven to 180°C.
2. After which you line a baking tray with baking paper and set aside.
3. After that, whisk eggs, honey, milk, and vanilla in a medium shallow dish.
4. Then, heat a large non-stick round frying pan over medium heat with spray olive oil.
5. Furthermore, dip 2 bread slices into the egg mixture, ensuring they are well coated.
6. After that, add to the pan and cook for about 2-3 minutes each side or until golden brown.
7. At this point, transfer to a baking tray and keep warm in the oven.
8. Make sure you repeat with remaining bread and egg mixture.

9. In the meantime, combine sliced sultanas, banana and cinnamon in a small bowl and toss to combine.
10. In addition, place French Toast onto serving plates and top with fruit mix and yoghurt.
11. Finally, you garnish with extra cinnamon.

Banana, berry & oat smoothie

Ingredients

2 tablespoons of reduced fat Greek yoghurt

½ cup of frozen (or fresh) mixed berries

1 tablespoon of flaked coconut (to serve)

1½ cup of reduced fat milk

1 banana

½ cup of rolled oats

1 tablespoon of chia seeds (to serve)

Directions:

1. First, you place yoghurt, milk, banana, mixed berries and oats into a blender or food processor and blend until smooth.
2. Finally, you pour smoothie into two tall glasses and top with chia seeds and coconut before serving.

Bircher muesli with tropical fruit

Ingredients

1 pear (peeled, cored and grated)

½ teaspoon of ground cinnamon

150g reduced fat vanilla yoghurt

1 cup (about 250ml) reduced fat milk

2 passion fruit (pulp)

1 apple (peeled, cored and grated)

2 cups of rolled oats

1 cup (about 250ml) unsweetened pear juice

50g flaked almonds (toasted)

2 mangoes, peeled and chopped (NOTE: use frozen mango if not in season)

1 banana (sliced)

Directions:

1. First, put the rolled oats, pear, apple, cinnamon and pear juice in a bowl and mix to combine, allow to stand covered in the refrigerator for an hour.
2. After which you fold through the yoghurt and almonds.
3. Finally, spoon the muesli into individual bowls and serve topped with the milk, mango and banana then drizzle with passionfruit pulp.

Tip: If you want to toast the flaked almonds, I suggest you place in a small non-stick frypan over a medium-high heat and stir until lightly browned.

Blueberry chia pot

Ingredients

½ teaspoon of vanilla extract

1 apple (half chopped and half grated)

1 tablespoon of coconut flakes (to serve)

¾ cup of reduced fat milk

¼ cup of chia seeds

2 tablespoons of blueberries (fresh or frozen), to serve

Directions:

1. First, you combine vanilla extract, milk, chia seeds and grated apple in a medium-size bowl.
2. After which you spoon mixture into 2 small bowls or jars and refrigerate for at least 30 minutes or until mixture is set.
3. Finally, top with apple, blueberries and flaked coconut to serve.

Breakfast Burrito

Ingredients

¼ cup of reduced fat milk

Olive oil spray

1 green capsicum (about 220g), halved, seeded, thinly sliced lengthways

1 x 150g can of no added salt corn kernels (drained)

8 small corn tortillas (approx. 30g per tortilla)

8 eggs

¼ cup (about 30g) grated reduced fat mozzarella

1 small red capsicum (about 220g), halved, seeded, thinly sliced lengthways

12 mushrooms (about 400g), thinly sliced

3 medium tomatoes (about 450g), diced

Directions:

1. First, whisk eggs and milk in a large bowl.
2. After which you stir in cheese; set aside.
3. After that, heat a large non-stick frying pan over medium-high heat and lightly spray with olive oil.
4. Then you stir-fry red and green capsicum for about 4-5 minutes or until softened.
5. At this point, add mushroom and corn, cook, stirring for about 2-3 minutes.
6. Furthermore, reduce heat to low and add egg mix.
7. After which you stir gently with a wooden spoon for 2 minutes or until eggs are just set.

8. This is when you remove pan from heat.
9. In addition, heat the tortillas according to packet instructions. Evenly spread each tortilla with egg, and vegetable mix, plus the diced tomato.
10. Finally, roll up burrito style and serve.

Note: Optional extras include lime wedge, coarsely chopped coriander, freshly chopped chili or hot sauce.

Homemade baked beans

Ingredients

1 red onion (finely chopped)

900g canned no added salt cannellini or butter beans, drained, rinsed

5 large ripe tomatoes (finely diced)

3 teaspoons of fresh parsley (finely chopped)

1 tablespoon of apple cider vinegar

6 slices of multigrain bread (toasted, to serve)

Spray olive oil

4 garlic cloves (peeled, finely diced)

2 sage leaves (roughly torn)

2 tablespoons of no-added-salt tomato paste

½ cup of reduced salt vegetable stock

3 cups of baby spinach leaves

Directions:

1. First, spray a large non-stick frying pan with olive oil and set over medium-high heat.
2. After which you add red onion and garlic to the pan cook for about 1-2 minutes, or until just softened.
3. After that, add sage, tomato paste, cannellini beans, ripe tomatoes, parsley, vegetable stock and ¼ cup water and cook for 10-15 minutes, or until sauce is thick.
4. Then, stir in apple cider vinegar and baby spinach leaves and heat, stir occasionally for about 5-10 minutes.

5. Finally, serve baked beans with Multigrain toast.

Tips:

Remember, baked beans can be stored in a sealed container for 3-4 days in the fridge, or up to 6 months in the freezer.

Whole meal pancakes with winter fruits

Ingredients

Stewed Winter Fruits:

½ bunch rhubarb (trimmed and sliced)

1 teaspoon of water

2 medium Granny Smith apples (peeled, cored and cut into small pieces)

1 teaspoon of ground cinnamon

1 teaspoon of lemon juice

Pancakes:

2 cups of reduced fat milk

1 small sized bananas (mashed)

400g reduced fat Greek Yoghurt

2 cups of whole meal self-rising flour

1 egg (lightly beaten)

Spray olive oil

Directions:

1. First, place rhubarb, lemon juice apples, cinnamon and water in a medium saucepan.
2. After which you stir to combine.
3. After that, cover and bring to the boil.
4. Then, reduce heat to medium and simmer for about 10-12 minutes or until fruit is tender; set aside.

5. At this point, you place flour in a large mixing bowl.
6. Furthermore, make a well in the center.
7. After which in another smaller mixing bowl, combine milk, egg, and mashed banana.
8. After that, pour banana mixture into well and whisk until smooth.
9. This is when you spray a large, non-stick frying pan with oil.
10. In addition, heat over medium heat.
11. Then spoon ¼ cup of pancake mixture into the pan.
12. At this point, cook for 2-3 minutes or until bubbles appear.
13. Turn; cook for about 1 to 2 minutes on the other side and transfer to a plate and repeat with remaining mixture.
14. Finally, place pancakes on plates and top with stewed winter fruits and yoghurt.

Mushroom, feta and thyme omelet

Ingredients

100g (about 3) medium mushrooms, sliced

2 teaspoons of chopped fresh (or better still ½ teaspoon dried) thyme leaves

1 tablespoons of water

Cracked black pepper (to season)

2 teaspoons of olive oil

1 tablespoon of semi-dried tomatoes, drained on paper towel, finely chopped

2 medium eggs

20g reduced fat feta cheese

Directions:

1. First, you heat 1 teaspoon of the oil in a small non-stick frypan.
2. After which you add mushrooms, sauté until tender then stir in semi-dried tomatoes and thyme and transfer mixture to bowl.
3. After that, whisk eggs and water together in a bowl.
4. Then, heat another teaspoon of oil in the same frypan.
5. At this point, you pour egg mixture into heated frypan and cook over a medium heat, drawing edges of mixture toward center so that unset mixture flows to the edge of pan.
6. Furthermore, when omelet is almost set, I suggest you sprinkle sautéed mushroom mixture and crumbled feta over half the omelet, season with pepper, then flip unfilled side over filling.

7. In addition, stand over a low heat for a further minute to allow filling to heat through.
8. This is when you slide omelet onto a serving plate and serve straight away.

Porridge with stewed apples and chopped pecans

Ingredients

2 tablespoons of water

3 cups of reduced fat milk

1 teaspoon of ground cinnamon

4 medium Green Apples (peeled, cored and cut into small pieces)

2 ½ cups of Rolled Oats

200g reduced fat Greek yoghurt

2 tablespoons of pecans (roughly chopped)

Directions:

1. First, place apples and water in a large saucepan over medium-low heat.
2. After which you bring to the boil; reduce heat to low.
3. After that, simmer, covered, for about 8-10 minutes or until apple is tender; set aside.
4. Then, place rolled oats and milk in a large saucepan over medium heat.
5. Furthermore, you bring to the boil, stir with a wooden spoon, then boil for about 5-7 minutes until oats are thick and creamy.
6. At this point, remove from the heat and spoon into bowls.
7. Finally, top with stewed apples, yoghurt, chopped pecans and cinnamon.

Smashed avocado with eggs on multigrain

Ingredients

1 tablespoon of fresh mint (roughly chopped)

½ teaspoon of freshly ground pepper

250g cherry tomatoes (halved)

8 eggs (soft boiled)

Cracked pepper (to serve)

2 avocados (halved, stoned and roughly chopped)

1 teaspoon of lemon juice

60g reduced-fat feta cheese

½ red onion (finely chopped)

4 thick slices multigrain/grainy bread (to serve)

Directions:

1. First, place mint, avocado, lemon juice and pepper in a small bowl and roughly mash with a fork.
2. After which you add feta, cherry tomatoes and red onion and toss lightly; set aside.

To soft boil an egg:

3. First, fill a medium-size saucepan with water and bring to the boil.
4. After that, gently place eggs in boiling water and boil for about 6-7 minutes.
5. Then you gently remove from pot and when cool to the touch, shell the egg, slice in half.
6. At this point, while eggs are boiling, toast bread.
7. This is when you divide the avocado smash and multigrain toast between the 4 plates.

8. Finally, top each with 2 eggs and finish with cracked pepper.

Tip: remember, poached eggs are a delicious alternative for this dish.

Smashed banana on fruit bread

Ingredients

4 medium sized bananas

480g reduced fat ricotta

2 tablespoons of honey

8 slices whole meal fruit toast (thinly sliced)

2 teaspoons of cinnamon

20 strawberries (washed, hulled and diced)

Directions:

1. First, in a bowl, cinnamon, mash together banana, and ricotta; set aside.
2. After which you toast fruit toast.
3. After that, spread the banana mixture evenly over the toast.
4. Then, evenly scatter diced strawberries over the banana mixture.
5. Finally, drizzle over honey and serve.

Delectable Salad and sides recipes

Warm roasted vegetable salad

Ingredients

2 zucchinis (halved lengthways, thickly sliced)

3 tablespoons of olive oil

150g of cherry tomatoes

1 teaspoon of baby capers (drained, chopped)

1 teaspoon of Dijon Mustard

25g reduced fat feta cheese

400g sweet potato (cut into 2cm pieces)

1 red onion (peeled and sliced into 6 chunks)

1 teaspoon of dried oregano

3 large flat mushrooms (sliced into chunks)

1 tablespoon of lemon juice

1 bunch parsley (roughly chopped)

50g spinach leaves

Directions:

1. Meanwhile, heat oven to 200°C.
2. After which you place zucchini, sweet potato, and red onion on a lined baking tray, drizzle with 1 tablespoon olive oil and dried oregano.
3. After that, roast for 20 minutes.

4. Then, add tomatoes and mushrooms on the tray and drizzle with 1 tablespoon olive oil, then return to the oven for a further 10-12 minutes until vegetables are tender and golden.
5. For the dressing, I suggest you whisk capers, Dijon mustard, lemon juice and remaining 1 tablespoon olive oil.
6. Furthermore, in a large bowl, gently toss roasted vegetables, parsley, and spinach leaves.
7. Finally, add the feta and dressing and toss gently.
8. Make sure you serve warm.

Warm roasted cauliflower, broccoli, walnut & lentil salad

Ingredients

8 broccoli florets

1 tablespoon of olive oil

3 tablespoons of walnuts (roughly chopped)

2 tablespoons of parsley (roughly chopped)

2 tablespoons of lemon juice

½ red onion (cut into chunks)

8 cauliflower florets

1 tablespoon of cumin

200g no-added-salt brown lentils (drained and rinsed)

2 tablespoons of mint (roughly chopped)

Directions:

1. Meanwhile, heat oven to 180°C.
2. After which you line a large baking tray with baking paper.
3. After that, place red onion, broccoli and cauliflower onto the baking tray; drizzle with olive oil and cumin.
4. Then you roast in the oven for about 20-25 minutes or until tender and vegetables are slightly charred.
5. At this point, add walnuts for the last 5 minutes of roasting.
6. Finally, place mint, lemon juice, lentils, parsley, walnuts and roasted vegetables into a bowl and toss to combine.
7. Make sure you serve warm.

Zucchini pasta salad

Ingredients

2 tablespoons of olive oil

60g black pitted olives

150g baby rocket

30g sundried tomatoes

1 tablespoon of lemon juice

1 garlic clove (minced)

200g penne pasta

1 x 250g punnet cherry tomatoes (halved)

2 spring onions (chopped)

1 small yellow capsicum (thinly sliced)

2 medium zucchinis (peeled into thin ribbons with a vegetable peeler)

¼ teaspoon of cracked pepper

Directions:

1. First, boil penne pasta in a large saucepan of boiling water following packet directions.
2. After which you drain, cool and place in a large salad bowl.
3. After that, add 1 tablespoon olive oil to cooled pasta; toss to combine.
4. At this point, add olives, capsicum, spring onion, cherry tomatoes, rocket, sundried tomatoes and zucchini; toss to combine.

To make dressing:

1. First, whisk together remaining lemon juice, olive oil, cracked pepper and garlic.
2. Then, toss through pasta salad and serve.

Warm roasted pumpkin dip with vegetable crudités & whole meal pita

Ingredients

2 tablespoons of olive oil

¼ teaspoon of cracked pepper

2 tablespoons of coriander leaves (roughly chopped)

1 small round whole meal pitas (cut into small triangles)

400g pumpkin (peeled, deseeded, diced)

2 teaspoons of cumin

¼ cup of reduced fat Greek yoghurt

2 medium carrots (peeled and cut into small batons)

4 sticks celery (cut into small batons)

Directions:

1. Meanwhile, heat oven to 180°C.
2. After which you place pumpkin on a lined baking tray, drizzle with 2 tablespoons olive oil.
3. After that, roast for 20-25 minutes or until golden and cooked.
4. Then, place pumpkin, cracked pepper, cumin, yoghurt and coriander leaves into a food processor.
5. Furthermore, process until a smooth dip form.
6. At this point, spoon into a small serving bowl.
7. Finally, serve with vegetable crudités and whole meal pita triangles.

Three pea stir-fries

Ingredients

2 teaspoons of honey

1 tablespoon of canola, sunflower or peanut oil

150g snow peas (topped and tailed)

1 garlic clove (crushed)

1 tablespoon of sesame seeds (toasted)

1 teaspoon of salt reduced soy sauce

1 teaspoon of sesame oil

150g sugar snap peas (trimmed)

2 teaspoons of cold water

1 tablespoon of finely grated fresh ginger

1 cup of frozen or fresh green peas

Directions:

1. First, combine the honey, soy sauce and sesame oil in a small jug, set aside.
2. After which you heat a wok over a high heat until hot.
3. After that, add the oil and swirl to coat the surface.
4. Then, add the snow peas, sugar snap peas, garlic and ginger and stir-fry for 1 minute.
5. Furthermore, add the fresh or frozen peas and 2 teaspoons of cold water.
6. At this point, toss to combine then quickly cover the wok and allow to stand for 15 seconds.
7. This is when you remove the lid, pour over the soy mixture and stir-fry 15 seconds.

8. Finally, remove from the heat scatter over the sesame seeds and serve.

Tip: remember, this stir-fry is a perfect accompaniment for lean beef or chicken, I suggest you serve with steamed rice.

Warm roasted cauliflower salad

Ingredients

3 tablespoons of olive oil

3 cups of rocket

1kg cauliflower (trimmed and cut into florets)

2 red onions (chopped into medium sized wedges)

1/3 cup of almonds (chopped)

Dressing:

2 tablespoons of lemon juice

1 tablespoon of parsley

2 tablespoons of tahini

4 tablespoons of warm water

Directions:

1. Meanwhile, heat oven to 180°C.
2. After which you place cauliflower on a lined baking tray, drizzle with 2 tablespoons olive oil.
3. After that, roast for about 20-25 minutes or until golden and cooked.
4. Then on a separate lined baking tray, place wedges of red onion and almonds.
5. At this point, drizzle with 1 tablespoon olive oil and roast for about 10-15 minutes or until golden.

To make dressing:

1. First, combine lemon juice, tahini, warm water and parsley and whisk to combine.
2. After which in a large salad bowl gently toss roasted cauliflower, almonds, red onion, and rocket and drizzle with dressing. Serve warm.

Warm asparagus and capsicum quinoa salad

Ingredients

2 cups (about 500ml) water

1 tablespoon of sunflower oil

2 cups of sliced spring onions

2 cloves garlic

1 tablespoon of salt reduced soy sauce and lime wedges, to serve

2/3 cup of quinoa

1 tablespoon (about 20g) Flora pro-active Original or Buttery

1 red capsicum

2 bunches asparagus (trimmed and sliced)

¼ cup of chopped parsley

2 tablespoons of chopped dill

Directions:

1. First, place quinoa and water in a saucepan over a medium heat and bring to the boil.
2. After which you reduce heat and simmer for 15 minutes (make sure you drain any excess water).
3. After that, heat Flora pro-active and oil in a wok over high heat.
4. Then add capsicum and cook, stirring for 2 minutes.
5. At this point, add the onions, asparagus and garlic and cook, stirring, just until the onion and asparagus are bright green.
6. Furthermore, stir in the quinoa, parsley and dill.
7. Finally, serve with lime wedges and a dash of soy sauce.

Avocado caprese salad

Ingredients

1½ tomatoes (thickly sliced)

¼ reduced fat mozzarella or bocconcini ball (roughly 100g), thinly sliced

½ teaspoon of freshly cracked black pepper

2 cups of rocket

½ avocado (cut into thin sliced)

4 tablespoons of basil leaves (roughly chopped)

1 tablespoon of olive oil

Directions:

First, spread rocket over the bottom of a serving platter.

After which you overlap the tomato, avocado and mozzarella on top of the rocket.

Then, scatter over basil leaves, then drizzle with olive oil and a sprinkle of pepper.

Faro with broad bean & pea salad

Ingredients

1 cup of broad beans (shelled)

3 tablespoons of mint (roughly chopped)

6 radishes (thinly sliced)

2 tablespoons of olive oil

50g reduced fat feta

1 cup faro (rinsed and drained)

1 cup of frozen peas

1 tablespoon of parsley (roughly chopped)

2 cups of rocket

1 tablespoon of lemon juice

Directions:

1. First, combine faro with 3 cups water in a medium saucepan.
2. After which you bring to the boil, then lower heat and simmer for about 20-30 minutes until faro is tender.
3. After that, drain well and transfer to a large bowl to cool.
4. Then, while faro is cooking, cook the broad beans and peas in a pot of boiling water for 3 minutes, then drain and refresh under cold water.
5. Finally, once faro has cooled, add broad beans, parsley, radishes, peas, mint, and rocket and toss gently to combine.

To prepare the dressing:

1. First, combine olive oil and lemon juice in a small bowl.
2. Then, pour dressing over salad and toss to combine.

3. Finally, sprinkle fetta over salad before serving.

Red potato salad

Ingredients

¾ cup of reduced fat Greek Yoghurt

½ tablespoon of Dijon mustard

2 tablespoons dill (roughly chopped)

2 spring onions (thinly sliced)

4 large red potatoes (skin on)

1 tablespoon of wholegrain mustard

1 small red onion (thinly sliced)

3 stalks celery (chopped)

Directions:

1. First, bring a large pot of water to the boil.
2. After which you add potatoes and cook until tender, approximately 15 minutes, drain.
3. After that, set aside to cool in a large salad bowl.
4. Then, in a small bowl combine wholegrain mustard, Greek yoghurt, Dijon mustard and dill; stir well to combine.
5. At this point, add celery, red onion, spring onion and dressing to the potatoes and stir gently to combine.
6. Finally, refrigerate for at least an hour before serving.

Roasted carrots with tahini yoghurt

Ingredients

1 tablespoon of olive oil

1 ½ teaspoons of ground cumin

½ teaspoon of cracked pepper

1 ½ tablespoons of coriander leaves (roughly chopped)

1 tablespoon of honey

1 tablespoon of ground coriander

3 thyme sprigs

8 carrots (peeled and cut into small batons)

Tahini Yoghurt Sauce:

130g reduced fat Greek Yoghurt

1 garlic clove (crushed)

40g tahini paste

2 tablespoons of lemon juice

Directions:

Meanwhile, heat oven to 200°C.

After which you spray a large rectangle baking tray with olive oil and line a large baking tray with baking paper.

For the Tahini Yoghurt Sauce:

1. First, whisk tahini paste, lemon juice, Greek yoghurt, and garlic in a small bowl and set aside.

2. After which you place the oil, honey, ground cumin, ground coriander, thyme and cracked pepper in a large mixing bowl.
3. Then add the carrots and mix well until coated then spread them out on prepared baking tray.
4. At this point, roast in the oven for about 40 minutes, stirring gently once or twice, until cooked through and glazed.
5. This is when you transfer the carrots to a large serving platter.
6. Finally, serve warm or at room temperature, with a spoonful of sauce on top and scatter with fresh coriander.

Potato bake

Ingredients

1 large red onion (halved, thinly sliced)

¼ cup of reduced fat thickened cream

2 teaspoons seeded (or Dijon mustard)

1.5kg unpeeled desire or Pontiac potatoes, thinly sliced

Fresh basil leaves

Olive oil spray

1 broccoli floret (chopped)

1 cup of reduced salt vegetable (or chicken stock)

Cracked black pepper (to season)

½ cup of reduced fat grated tasty cheese

Directions:

1. Meanwhile, heat oven to 220°C (200°C fan-forced).
2. After which you lightly grease a 3cm x 20cm ovenproof dish with cooking spray.
3. After that, place onions and broccoli onto a microwave-safe bowl; lightly spray with oil.
4. Then you cover loosely with paper towel and microwave on high for 5 minutes or until soft.
5. At this point, whisk the stock, cream, mustard and black pepper together in a jug until well combined.
6. Furthermore, arrange 1/3 of the potatoes over the base of the dish.
7. This is when you top with half the onion and broccoli then pour over half the stock mixture; repeat the layers.

8. In addition, cover with a piece of baking paper then foil and bake for 1 hour or until potatoes are tender.

9. After that, remove the paper and foil, lightly spray with cooking oil and scatter over the cheese and basil (if using).

10. Finally, increase oven to 250°C (230°C fan-forced) and bake uncovered for a further 15 minutes or until lightly golden.

Moroccan herb couscous

Ingredients

2 teaspoons of ground cumin

1 teaspoon of paprika

1 teaspoon of orange zest

1 medium red capsicum (thinly sliced)

3 cups of baby spinach leaves (roughly chopped)

¼ cup of pepitas

2 tablespoons of olive oil

½ cup of uncooked whole meal couscous

½ teaspoon of ground ginger

1 orange

1 medium zucchini (peeled into thin ribbons with a vegetable peeler)

5 radishes (thinly sliced)

½ cup of raisins

3 tablespoons parsley (roughly chopped)

3 tablespoons mint (roughly chopped)

Directions:

1. First, cook couscous according to packet instructions; set aside.
2. Then, once couscous is cooled, transfer the couscous to a large bowl and add ginger, cumin, and paprika power, using a fork to gently loosen up the couscous to ensure there are no clumps.

3. After which you grate the zest of the orange before slicing the orange into small wedges ensuring to remove any white pith.
4. After that, add to the bowl.
5. Finally, add red capsicum, zucchini, parsley, radishes, raisins, spinach, pepitas, mint and olive oil.
6. Then toss to combine and serve.

Pesto pumpkin salad

Ingredients

Spray olive oil

200g rocket leaves

40g low fat feta cheese (crumbled)

500g butternut pumpkin (peeled, seeds removed, cut into small cubes)

50g pine nuts

150g cherry tomatoes (halved)

1 red onion (finely diced)

Pesto:

½ bunch of fresh basil

1 tablespoon of parmesan cheese

1 teaspoon of lemon juice

½ clove garlic

1 tablespoon of pine nuts

2 tablespoon of olive oil

Directions:

1. Meanwhile, heat oven to 180°C.
2. After which you line 1 baking tray with baking paper.
3. After that, place pumpkin on baking tray and spray with olive oil.
4. Then roast, turning once, for 30 minutes or until golden and tender, set aside.

In the meantime, to make pesto,

1. First, place the pine nuts, parmesan cheese, garlic, basil, and lemon juice in a food processor and process until finely chopped; with the motor running, gradually add in olive oil until well combined; set aside
2. Then, in a large bowl, toss the rocket, pine nuts, cherry tomatoes, red onion and pumpkin.
3. Finally, add the feta and pesto and toss gently.

Lemony green salad with radicchio & pepitas

Ingredients

- 3 cups of baby spinach leaves
- ½ head radicchio (cored and sliced)
- 1 tablespoon of lemon juice
- 2 tablespoons of shaved parmesan
- ½ cup of pepitas
- 3 cups of rocket leaves
- 2 tablespoons of lemon zest
- 3 tablespoons of olive oil
- 1 teaspoon of honey

Directions:

1. Meanwhile, heat oven to 200°C.
2. After which you place pepitas on a prepared baking tray and bake for 5-8 minutes or until roasted; set aside to cool.
3. Then, in a large bowl, toss rocket, spinach leaves, radicchio, and pepitas.

To make the dressing:

1. First, combine lemon juice, lemon zest, olive oil and honey and whisk until slightly thickened.
2. Then you mix dressing through the salad and sprinkle shaved parmesan over the top before serving.

Tip: Remember, roasted red onion can also be added for some variety.

Delectable recipes for Lunch

Paprika chicken with pumpkin and spinach salad

Ingredients

1 garlic clove (crushed)

4 small skinless chicken breast fillets (about 450g), trimmed

1 tablespoon of smoked paprika

1 lemon (rind finely grated, juiced)

Pumpkin & spinach salad:

Olive oil cooking spray

1 small orange (juiced)

1 teaspoon of honey

100g baby spinach leaves

750g butternut pumpkin (cut into 2cm pieces)

Black pepper (to season)

1 tablespoon of extra virgin olive oil

Pinch ground cinnamon

Directions:

For the pumpkin & spinach salad:

1. Meanwhile, heat oven to 240°C (220°C fan-forced).
2. After which you line a large baking tray with non-stick baking paper.
3. After that, place the pumpkin on the tray.

4. Then, spray with olive oil and season with pepper.
5. At this point, roast for about 15-20 minutes or until golden and tender; set aside to cool to room temperature.
6. In the meantime, combine, garlic, paprika, lemon rind and juice in a shallow ceramic dish.
7. This is when you add chicken and turn to coat.
8. Furthermore, cover and refrigerate for about 10 minutes if time permits.
9. Meanwhile, heat barbecue plate on medium heat.
10. In addition, remove the chicken from the marinade.
11. After which you place a piece baking paper onto the hot barbecue plate and top with chicken.
12. After that, barbecue for 5-6 minutes each side or until cooked through.
13. At this point, transfer to a plate, cover and allow to rest for 5 minutes; discard the paper.
14. Then whisk the oil, orange juice, honey and cinnamon together.
15. Finally, combine the spinach and pumpkin in a bowl; spoon over the dressing and toss gently to combine.
16. Make sure you serve with the paprika chicken.

Moroccan spiced fish with couscous and raisin salad

Ingredients

2 teaspoons of ground cumin

1 garlic clove (crushed)

1 lemon (rind finely grated and juiced)

Olive oil spray

1 teaspoon of ground turmeric

2 teaspoons of ground coriander

2 teaspoons of olive oil

600g boneless fish fillets, skin on (snapper, ling or blue trevalla)

Couscous salad:

¼ cup of raisins (finely chopped)

¼ cup of pine nuts (toasted)

1 green capsicum (finely diced)

350g baby rocket

Lemon wedges (to serve)

0.5 cup of couscous

¼ cup of craisins

3 spring onions (finely chopped)

½ cup of fresh bean sprouts (trimmed)

1 cup of roughly chopped coriander leaves

Cracked black pepper (to season)

Directions:

1. First, combine the cumin, coriander, turmeric, garlic and oil in a shallow ceramic dish.
2. After which you add the lemon rind and 2 tablespoons of the juice, mix well.
3. After that, coat both sides of the fish fillets in the spice mixture.
4. Then you cover and refrigerate for up to 30 minutes, but no longer.

For the couscous salad:

1. First, place the couscous in a large heatproof bowl.
2. After which you pour over 1 cup boiling water.
3. After that, cover and set aside for 5-10 minutes or until couscous has absorbed the water.
4. Then you combine the craisins, green onions, raisins, pine nuts, bean sprouts, capsicum, rocket and coriander in a large bowl.
5. Furthermore, pour the remaining lemon juice over the couscous and fluff the grains with a fork.
6. At this point, add the raisin mixture, season with pepper and toss to combine.
7. This is when you heat a large non-stick frying pan or barbecue flat-plate on medium heat.
8. Spray lightly with oil; cook the fish fillets for 2-3 minutes each side, depending on thickness until golden and cooked through.
9. In addition, transfer to a plate, cover and allow to rest for 3 minutes.
10. Finally, spoon the couscous salad onto serving plates and top with the fish.
11. You can serve with lemon.

Grilled chicken salad bowl with tahini dressing

Ingredients

- 1 garlic clove (crushed)
- Olive oil spray
- 1 teaspoon of honey
- 200g can of no added salt lentils (drained)
- 2 large carrots (peeled, grated)
- 120g baby spinach
- 2 tablespoons of tahini
- 2 tablespoons of lemon juice
- 3 teaspoons of olive oil
- 400g lean chicken breasts (halved horizontally)
- 2 medium beetroots (peeled, grated)
- 1 large cucumber (cut into thick batons)

Directions:

1. First, combine garlic, lemon juice, tahini, olive oil and honey in a small bowl with 1 teaspoon hot water and mix until a smooth consistency; set aside.
2. After which you spray a large pan or non-stick frying pan with olive oil and heat over medium-high heat.
3. After that, cook chicken 5-6 minutes each side, or until golden and just cooked through; set aside.
4. If you want to serve, I suggest you divide the carrot, cucumber, lentils, beetroot, spinach leaves and sliced chicken between 4 bowls.
5. Finally, drizzle each bowl with tahini dressing.

Fish skewers with tabbouleh

Ingredients

1 orange (rind finely grated, juiced)

2 teaspoons of olive oil

3 pieces whole meal Lebanese bread

600g skinless firm white fish (like ling or barramundi), cut into 3cm cubes

2cm piece ginger (peeled, finely grated)

Olive oil spray

Tabbouleh:

¾ cup of burghul (cracked wheat)

1 cup of chopped fresh flat leaf parsley

½ cup of fresh mint leaves (chopped)

3 medium tomatoes (seeds removed, chopped)

3 spring onions (finely chopped)

1 tablespoon of olive oil

2 tablespoons of lemon juice

400g mixed green leaves

Directions:

To make the tabbouleh salad:

1. First, place burghul in a bowl.
2. After which you cover with boiling water; stand for 15 minutes or until softened.

3. After that, drain, pressing out all water using back of a large metal spoon then transfer to a large bowl.
4. Then add the remaining ingredients and stir to combine.
5. At this point, thread fish pieces onto eight small bamboo skewers.
6. Place in a shallow ceramic dish; combine juice, orange rind, ginger and olive oil in a jar, shake until well combined.
7. This is when you pour over fish; turn to coat.
8. In addition, cover and refrigerate for 15 minutes, if time permits.
9. Meanwhile, heat barbecue plate on medium-high heat and lightly spray with oil.
10. After that, remove the skewers from the marinade and barbecue, for about 6 minutes, turning or until fish is just cooked through.
11. Transfer to a plate; cover and stand for about 5 minutes.
12. Then, wrap Lebanese bread into foil and place on the barbecue for 5-6 minutes, to warm through.
13. Finally, place bread onto plates, top with tabbouleh salad and fish skewers.
14. You can serve with mixed green salad

Tip: remember, to soak skewers in cold water for at least 30 minutes before threading to avoid burning.

Falafel bowl

Ingredients

Falafels

3 cloves garlic

2 tablespoons of parsley

2 teaspoons of ground cumin

1 egg

Parsley salad

4 tomatoes (roughly chopped)

1 Lebanese cucumber (diced)

Tahini yoghurt

1 garlic clove (crushed)

1 tablespoon of lemon juice

¼ teaspoon of freshly ground black pepper

4 lemon wedges (to serve)

600g no-added-salt chickpeas (drained and rinsed)

1 brown onion (roughly chopped)

2 tablespoons of coriander

4 tablespoons of whole meal plain flour

2 tablespoons of olive oil

1 bunch parsley (roughly chopped)

1 red onion (finely chopped)

2 tablespoons of lemon juice

½ cup of reduced fat Greek yoghurt

2 tablespoons of tahini

½ teaspoon of ground cumin

1 tablespoon of olive oil

4 x small whole meal pita breads, to serve

Directions:

1. First, place garlic, parsley, cumin, chickpeas, onion, coriander, flour and egg into a food processor and process until almost smooth.
2. After which you use your hands, divide the mixture into 8 and roll 8 falafel patties.
3. After that, you cover and refrigerate for about 30-45 minutes.

In the meantime, **prepare parsley salad.**

A. At this point, combine tomatoes, parsley, red onion, cucumber, and lemon juice in a medium bowl and stir to combine; set aside.

To make tahini yoghurt:

a) First, you whisk together garlic, ground cumin, yoghurt, tahini, lemon juice, pepper and olive oil in a small bowl until well combined.
b) After which you heat oil in a large frying pan over medium heat.
c) After that, cook patties for about 4-5 minutes each side or until cooked through.
4. If you want to serve, divide the falafels, parsley salad, and pitas between the 4 bowls.
5. Finally, top with tahini yoghurt and a lemon wedge.

Chicken, rice and bean bowl

Ingredients

1 teaspoon of paprika

1 tablespoon of olive oil

250g green beans (trimmed)

2 cups of baby spinach

1 (250g) punnet cherry tomatoes, halved

4 lemon wedges (to serve)

1 teaspoon of lemon zest

¼ cup (about 60ml) lemon juice

8 chicken tenderloins (about 500g total)

2 cups '90 second quick' brown rice and quinoa blend

1 (425g) can black beans (rinsed, drained)

1 (300g) corn kernels (rinsed, drained)

Directions:

1. First, combine the paprika, zest, lime juice and olive oil in a ceramic dish.
2. After which you add the chicken and turn to coat; set aside.
3. After that, steam, boil or microwave the green beans for 2-3 minutes or until just tender; drain.
4. Then, heat a large chargrill pan or barbeque hotplate over medium heat.
5. At this point, grill the chicken for 3-4 minutes each side, or until cooked through.
6. In the meantime, heat microwave brown rice & quinoa blend according to packet instructions.

7. Furthermore, divide the brown rice & quinoa blend between the 4 bowls.
8. This is when you top each with black beans, spinach, tomatoes, corn kernels and 2 chicken tenderloins.
9. Finally, serve with a lemon wedge in each bowl.

Chicken and corn soup

Ingredients

6 spring onions (thinly sliced)

Pinch dried chili flakes

3 corn cobs, kernels removed

420g can creamed corn

250g dried egg noodles (optional)

2 x 200g skinless chicken breast fillets (trimmed of fat)

2 garlic cloves (crushed)

Olive oil spray

4 cups of reduced salt chicken stock

2 teaspoons of reduced salt soy sauce

Extra sliced spring onions (to serve)

Directions:

1. First, place chicken in a deep pan; cover with cold water.
2. After which you bring to the boil over medium heat.
3. After that, reduce the heat to low, then cover with a lid and simmer for 8 minutes.
4. Then you remove the pan from heat and set aside for 15 minutes.
5. At this point, drain the chicken then shred into pieces.
6. This is when you heat a saucepan over medium heat until hot and spray lightly with oil.
7. Furthermore, add the garlic, onions, and chili.
8. After which you cook, stirring often for 5 minutes or until soft.
9. Then, add the corn kernels and cook for 1 minute.

10.   In addition, pour in the stock and bring to the boil.
11. After that, add the chicken, creamed corn, and soy, cook 4-5 minutes until chicken is warmed through.
12. Finally, serve topped with extra spring onions of desired.

A handy tip: feel free to substitute frozen corn kernels for canned no added salt corn kernels (drained).

Chicken and salad wholegrain rolls

Ingredients

400g lean chicken breasts (halved horizontally)

¼ purple cabbage (trimmed, shredded)

1 large capsicum (seeded and finely diced)

3 tablespoons of mint (chopped)

4 wholegrain rolls

Spray olive oil

4 spring onions (finely sliced)

2 carrots (peeled and grated)

3 tablespoons of coriander (chopped)

2 tablespoons of sweet chili sauce

Directions:

1. First, you heat a large pan or non-stick frying pan over medium-high heat and spray with olive oil.
2. After which you cook chicken 5-6 minutes each side, or until golden and just cooked through; set aside.
3. In the meantime, to prepare Asian Slaw combine the red cabbage, carrots, capsicum, spring onion, coriander and mint in a large bowl.
4. After that, add sweet chili sauce to the Asian Slaw and toss to combine.
5. Then, place a chicken breast on each roll base and top with Asian Slaw and roll lid to serve.

Delectable recipe for Dinner

BBQ pork with cabbage and apple salad

Ingredients

1 tablespoon of honey

Olive oil spray

1 tablespoon of unsweetened apple juice

Cracked black pepper (to season)

½ cup of walnuts (toasted and roughly chopped)

1 tablespoon of wholegrain mustard

4 small (about 120g each) pork loin cutlets or medallions, trimmed of fat

2 tablespoons of low-fat natural Greek-style yoghurt

2 teaspoons of Dijon mustard

2 pink lady apples (cut into thin wedges)

¼ small (about 400g) green cabbage, finely shredded

Directions:

1. First, you combine the seeded mustard and honey together in a small bowl.
2. After which you brush over both sides of the pork.
3. Meanwhile, heat a barbecue plate or large non-stick frying pan over a medium heat.
4. After that, spray lightly with oil to grease.
5. Then add pork and cook for 3-5 minutes on each side, or until golden and just cooked through.
6. Finally, remove the pork to a plate and cover to keep warm.

For the salad:

1. First, whisk the apple juice, yoghurt, and mustard together in a medium size bowl until well combined.
2. After which you season with freshly ground black pepper.
3. Then, add the apple, cabbage and walnuts and toss to combine.
4. This is when you pile the salad onto plates, top with pork and serve.

Almond & oat crusted salmon with vegetable kebabs

Ingredients

1 tablespoon of rolled oats

1 tablespoon of fresh dill

1 teaspoon of lemon juice

Vegetable Kebabs

1 medium red capsicum (halved, seeded, cut into chunks)

½ red onion (cut into chunks)

2 cloves garlic (minced)

2 lemon wedges (to serve)

 2 x 100-120g salmon fillets

1 tablespoon of almonds

2 teaspoons of lemon zest

1 tablespoon of olive oil

6 Bamboo Skewers, soaked in water for 30 minutes

1 zucchini (cut into chunks)

6 cherry tomatoes

½ teaspoon of freshly cracked black pepper

Directions:

1. Meanwhile, heat oven to 180°C.
2. After which you line a small baking tray and a large baking tray with baking paper; set aside.

To prepare salmon crust:

1. First, place rolled oats, lemon zest, almonds, dill, lemon juice and olive oil in a mortar and pestle and pound until paste forms. (NOTE: If you don't have a mortar and pestle, I suggest a small food processor can be used instead).
2. After that, place salmon fillets onto prepared small baking tray and press crust on top.
3. Then, bake in the oven for about 10-15 minutes until salmon is cooked and crust is golden.

To prepare vegetable skewers:

1. First, place zucchini, cherry tomatoes, capsicum, red onion, garlic and pepper into a small bowl and toss to combine.
2. After which you thread the vegetables onto 4 skewers.
3. After that, place vegetable skewers onto the prepared large baking tray and bake in the oven for 10-15 minutes until vegetables are roasted and cooked through.
4. Finally, serve salmon with vegetable skewers and a lemon wedge.

Butter-less butter chicken

Ingredients

2 onions (finely diced)

1 tablespoon of grated fresh ginger

1 tablespoon of cumin

1 tablespoon of brown sugar

½ teaspoon of turmeric

400g can no added salt diced tomatoes

300g green beans (trimmed and steamed)

2 cups of cooked basmati rice (to serve)

1 tablespoon of canola oil

4 garlic cloves (crushed)

2 tablespoons of no added salt tomato paste

1 tablespoon of garam masala

½ teaspoon of dried chili flakes

2 (about 250g each) skinless chicken breast fillets, trimmed of all visible fat

¾ cup of reduced fat thick natural yoghurt

Coriander sprigs (to garnish)

1 tablespoon of toasted flaked almonds (to garnish)

Directions:

1. First, you heat oil in a deep non-stick frying pan over medium heat.

2. After which you add onion and cook for 10 minutes.
3. After that, add garlic and ginger, cook 2 minutes.
4. Then add tomato paste, cook 1 minute.
5. Furthermore, reduce heat to low and stir in the garam masala, brown sugar, cumin, chili flakes and turmeric.
6. At this point, cut the chicken into pieces and add to the pan; cook, stirring, for 2-3 minutes.
7. This is when you add the yoghurt, tomatoes, and ¼ cup water, stir to combine.
8. In addition, bring to the boil then reduce heat to low and cook, uncovered, for 15-20 minutes or until the chicken is cooked and the sauce has thickened.
9. After which you serve with cooked basmati rice and the steamed beans.
10. Finally, garnish with coriander sprigs and toasted flaked almonds.

Bolognese pasta bake

Ingredients

1 brown onion (finely chopped)

400g lean beef mince

2 carrots (grated)

Cracked black pepper (to season)

250g reduced fat ricotta cheese

Green salad (to serve)

1 tablespoon of olive oil

2 garlic cloves (crushed)

2 cups of tomato passata sauce

2 zucchini (grated)

250g dried macaroni pasta

½ cup of grated reduced fat mozzarella

Directions:

1. First, heat oil in a large non-stick frying pan over medium heat.
2. After which you add onion and garlic and cook, stirring occasionally, for 5 minutes or until soft.
3. After that, increase the heat to high and add the mince.
4. Then, cook, stirring with a wooden spoon to break up mince, for 10 minutes or until browned.
5. At this point, stir in the tomato passata sauce and bring to the boil.
6. This is when you reduce heat to medium and add carrots and zucchini.

7. Furthermore, you simmer, uncovered, for 8-10 minutes or until the sauce thickens slightly.
8. After which you season with freshly ground black pepper.
9. Meanwhile, heat oven to 220°C (200°C fan-forced).
10. In the meantime, cook the pasta in a large saucepan of unsalted boiling water, following packet directions until al dente.
11. In addition, drain pasta and stir into the mince mixture.
12. After that, spoon mixture into one 8 cup capacity ovenproof dish or four 2 cup capacity individual ovenproof ramekins.
13. Then, crumble over the ricotta, then sprinkle with mozzarella.
14. Finally, bake for 20 minutes or until golden and bubbling around the edges.
15. Then serve with green salad.

Beef stroganoff

Ingredients

¼ cup plain flour

1 onion (peeled and sliced)

250g button mushrooms (sliced)

1 tablespoon of Worcestershire sauce

Black pepper (to season)

Mashed potato and steamed greens (to serve)

500g beef stir fry strips (trimmed of all visible fat)

2 tablespoons of olive oil

2 cloves garlic (peeled and crushed)

1 cup of salt reduced beef stock

1/3 cup of light sour cream

2 tablespoons of roughly chopped parsley

Directions:

1. First, coat the beef strips with the flour, discard any leftover flour.
2. After which you heat half the oil in a deep-frying pan and cook the beef over high heat in two batches until just cooked through.
3. After that, remove from pan, and set aside.
4. Then, add remaining oil to pan and cook the garlic, onion and mushrooms.
5. At this point, return beef to pan, pour in beef stock and Worcestershire.
6. Furthermore, bring to boil and simmer until sauce thickens slightly.

7. This is when you stir through sour cream, season with pepper.
8. Finally, sprinkle with parsley and serve with mashed potato and steamed greens.

Beef rissoles

Ingredients

1 small onion (peeled and finely chopped)

¼ red capsicum (finely chopped)

2 tablespoons of plain flour

Black pepper (to season)

Leafy green salad (to serve)

750g lean minced beef

2 Roma tomatoes (finely chopped)

2 tablespoons of dried mixed herbs

2 medium eggs (lightly beaten)

1 tablespoon of canola oil

Directions:

1. First, combine the onion, beef, tomatoes, herbs, capsicum, flour and eggs in a bowl.
2. After which you mix well, season with pepper.
3. After that, divide mixture into 12 equal portions, shape into rissoles.
4. Then place on baking tray lined with baking paper and refrigerate for 15 minutes.
5. Furthermore, you heat half the oil in a large frying pan over medium heat and cook rissoles in two batches.
6. At this point, cook rissoles for about 4-5 minutes each side or until golden and just cooked through.
7. In addition, heat remaining oil to cook second batch.
8. Finally, serve with leafy green salad.

Beef and green vegetable pasta bake

Ingredients

2 garlic cloves (finely chopped)

1 green capsicum (halved, seeded, thinly sliced length-ways)

1 x 400g can no-added-salt chopped tomatoes

250g whole meal penne pasta

4 tablespoons of shaved parmesan

1 tablespoon of olive oil

400g lean beef (mince)

500g vine-ripened tomatoes (coarsely chopped)

2 cups of baby spinach

1 bunch broccolini (trimmed and chopped)

2 cups of green beans (trimmed and chopped)

Directions:

1. Meanwhile, heat oven to 200°C.
2. After which you lightly grease a large deep baking tray.
3. After that, add olive oil to a large non-stick frying pan and set over medium-high heat.
4. Then, add onion and garlic to the pan cook for 1-2 minutes, or until just softened.
5. Furthermore, add beef mince and capsicum and cook, stirring, for 2 minutes or until browned.
6. At this point, add all tomatoes and bring to the boil.
7. This is when you reduce heat to low and simmer for 5-8 minutes or until sauce thickens.

8. In addition, stir through spinach leaves; while meat sauce is simmering, cook pasta in boiling water until al dente.
9. After that, add broccolini and green beans for the last minute of cooking time; drain.
10. Then stir pasta and green vegetables through tomato sauce.
11. This is the point where you add pasta-green vegetable mix to prepared baking tray and sprinkle with shaved parmesan.
12. Finally, grill for 5 minutes or until cheese is golden.
13. Serve.

Chicken & mushroom pot pies with steamed greens and baby potatoes

Ingredients

2 tablespoons of olive oil

2 small leeks (sliced)

300g button mushrooms (sliced)

1 ½ cups of reduced fat milk

4 sheets Filo Pastry

2 bunches broccolini (trimmed)

Spray olive oil

400g lean chicken breast (cut into 1cm pieces)

2 cloves garlic (crushed)

¼ cup of whole meal plain flour

½ teaspoon of cracked black pepper

1 egg (lightly beaten)

8 baby potatoes

Directions:

1. Meanwhile, heat oven to 200°C.
2. After which you spray 4 medium sized ramekins or oven dishes with olive oil.
3. After that, place a medium heavy based pan over medium heat and add 1 tablespoon olive oil.
4. Then, add the chicken and cook for 10-12 minutes or until cooked.
5. At this point, remove meat from the pot and set aside.

6. This is when you add remaining olive oil to the pan and sauté leeks, garlic and mushrooms for 5-6 minutes, or until just softened.
7. Furthermore, add the flour and cook for 1-2 minutes.
8. After that, add the milk and black pepper and cook for a further 4-5 minutes or until thickened.
9. In addition, return the chicken to the pot and stir to combine.
10. After which you refrigerate mixture until cooled completely.
11. In the meantime, bring a medium sized pot of water to the boil.
12. Then add potatoes and cook until tender, approximately 15 minutes, drain.
13. At this point, bring a small pan of water to the boil
14. This is when you add the broccolini and simmer for 4 minutes until tender; drain.
15. Meanwhile, once chicken mixture has cooled, divide chicken mixture between ramekins/oven dishes.
16. Finally, roughly press down 1 piece of filo on top of every ramekin and brush with egg.
17. Bake for 20 minute or until golden; serve with steamed greens and potatoes.

Chili fish stir fry

Ingredients

2 garlic cloves (crushed)

460g blue-eye trevalla or other firm white fish (cut into 3cm pieces)

200g snow peas (trimmed, sliced diagonally)

4 green onions (sliced)

1 tablespoon of salt-reduced soy sauce

2 tablespoons of fresh coriander for garnish

2 tablespoons of olive oil

1 tablespoon of fresh ginger (grated)

220g Hokkien noodles

1 bunch broccolini (sliced)

1 bunch baby bok choy (chopped)

1 ½ tablespoons of sweet chili sauce

¼ teaspoon of chili flakes

Directions:

1. First, heat oil in a non-stick frying pan over medium-high heat.
2. After which you cook garlic, ginger and fish, stirring occasionally, until fish is almost cooked through.
3. After that, transfer to a plate and set aside.
4. Then, cook or heat noodles according to packet instructions; drain well.
5. At this point, add broccolini, snow peas and green onion to the pan, cook for 2-3 minutes or until tender.

6. Furthermore, add soy sauce, bok choy, noodles, sweet chili sauce and chili flakes.
7. This is when you cook, stirring for another 2 minutes until noodles are heated through.
8. In addition, return cooked fish to the pan and cook stirring for 1 minute.
9. Finally, garnish with fresh coriander.

Chicken parmigiana

Ingredients

1 brown onion (finely diced)

1 eggplant (finely diced)

400g can no-added-salt chopped tomatoes

3 cups of baby spinach leaves

½ cup of reduced fat mozzarella cheese (grated)

Basil leaves (to serve)

4 x 120-150g skinless chicken breast fillets

1 clove garlic (crushed)

310g jar roasted pepper strips (drained)

2 tomatoes (roughly chopped)

1 cup of basil leaves (roughly chopped)

½ cup of fresh breadcrumbs

4 cups of green beans (trimmed)

Directions:

1. Meanwhile, heat oven to 200°C.
2. In the meantime, heat a non-stick frying pan on high heat.
3. After which you cook chicken breast for 3-4 minutes on each side or until cooked through.
4. After that, transfer to a plate and cover to keep warm.
5. In the meantime, using the same pan, add garlic, onion, eggplant and roasted red pepper strips and cook, stirring occasionally for 3-4 minutes until softened.
6. Then add chopped and fresh tomatoes and simmer for 4-5 minutes until sauce thickens.

7. At this point, add spinach and basil leaves and remove from the heat.
8. Furthermore, put cooked chicken breast onto a deep baking tray.
9. This is when you top with sauce and sprinkle with cheese and breadcrumbs.
10. In addition, bake for 10-15 minutes or until top is golden.
11. Then, while cooking, cook green beans in a saucepan of boiling water for 4-5 minutes or until just tender; drain.
12. Finally, serve Chicken with Green Beans and garnish with fresh basil leaves.

Delectable Snacks and dessert recipes

Warm roasted pumpkin dip with vegetable crudités & whole meal pita

Ingredients

2 tablespoons of olive oil

¼ teaspoon of cracked pepper

2 tablespoons of coriander leaves (roughly chopped)

1 small round whole meal pitas (cut into small triangles)

400g pumpkin (peeled, deseeded, diced)

2 teaspoons of cumin

¼ cup of reduced fat Greek yoghurt

2 medium carrots (peeled and cut into small batons)

4 sticks celery (cut into small batons)

Directions:

1. Meanwhile, heat oven to 180°C.
2. After which you place pumpkin on a lined baking tray, drizzle with 2 tablespoons olive oil.
3. After that, roast for 20-25 minutes or until golden and cooked.
4. Then, place cumin, pumpkin, cracked pepper, yoghurt and coriander leaves into a food processor.
5. Furthermore, process until a smooth dip form.
6. At this point, spoon into a small serving bowl.
7. Finally, you serve with vegetable crudités and whole meal pita triangles.

Spinach hummus with Turkish toasts

Ingredients

Olive oil spray

2 cups (about 60g) baby spinach leaves

2 tablespoons of tahini (sesame seed paste)

1 teaspoon of ground cumin

Raw vegetable pieces (e.g. celery, cucumber, carrot, beans), to serve

1 x loaf (about 430g) Turkish bread

1 x 400g can chick peas (rinsed and drained)

1 clove garlic (chopped)

¼ cup of lemon juice

2 tablespoons water (approximately)

Freshly cracked black pepper (to season)

Directions:

1. First, cut Turkish bread into 1cm thick slices and spray with cooking spray.
2. After which you toast slices under a preheated grill, char-grill pan or barbecue until crisp and lightly browned on both sides.
3. After that, process chick peas, spinach and garlic in a food processor until finely chopped.
4. Then, add lemon juice, tahini, cumin and water and process again until smooth.

5. At this point, transfer mixture to a bowl and season with pepper. (**NOTE:** if consistency is too thick, I suggest you stir in a little extra water).
6. Then serve dip with Turkish toasts and vegetable pieces.

Savory muffins

Ingredients

1 medium zucchini grated

¼ cup of frozen peas

1 red capsicum (finely chopped)

1 tablespoon of chives (finely chopped)

½ cup of reduced fat milk

2 tablespoons of olive oil

3 teaspoons of baking powder

Spray olive oil

1 medium carrot (grated)

¼ cup of frozen corn

1 tablespoon of parsley (finely chopped)

½ cup of reduced fat cheddar cheese, grated

¼ cup of reduced fat Greek yoghurt

2 eggs

2 cups of whole meal plain flour

Directions:

1. Meanwhile, heat oven to 180°C.
2. After which you spray 8 large muffin hole tray with olive oil and set aside.
3. After that, place the grated zucchini and carrot into either a sieve or a clean tea towel and squeeze out the juice.

4. Then, place the carrot, zucchini, peas, capsicum, chives, milk, corn, parsley, cheese, yoghurt and egg in a large mixing bowl and stir until combined.

5. Furthermore, add flour and baking powder to wet ingredients and fold in gently until just combined.

6. At this point, spoon the mixture evenly between 8 muffin holes.

7. In addition, bake for 20-25 minutes or until golden and mixture is set.

8. Finally, once defrosted, muffins can be enjoyed cold or warmed in the oven.

Salmon, ricotta and quinoa cups (gluten free)

Ingredients

1/3 cup of quinoa

1 fresh corn cob (husk removed)

200g reduced fat ricotta cheese

1 cup of grated zucchini (1 small-medium)

¾ cup of grated reduced fat tasty cheese

Canola or olive oil spray

2/3 cup of water

6 large eggs

1 x 210g can red salmon (drained and flaked)

2 spring onions (thinly sliced)

Directions:

1. First, grease a 12-hole (1/3 cup capacity) non-stick or silicone muffin tray with spray oil.
2. Meanwhile, heat oven to 190°C (170°C fan-forced).
3. After which you place quinoa and water in a small saucepan; bring to boil.
4. After that, reduce heat, simmer covered for about 10 minutes or until all liquid has been absorbed; remove.
5. Then, stand covered for 10 minutes.
6. At this point, cut corn kernels from the cob.
7. Furthermore, whisk the eggs and ricotta in a large bowl until combined.
8. This is when you stir in corn, zucchini, quinoa, salmon, shallots and grated cheese.

9. At this point, spoon mixture evenly into muffin tray.
10. In addition, bake in preheated oven for 20-25 minutes or until set and light golden.
11. Finally, stand quinoa cups in muffin tray 10 minutes, then loosen edges and remove.

Salmon & polenta pikelets

Ingredients

½ cup of boiling water

2 tablespoons of reduced fat milk

2 tablespoons of reduced fat cottage cheese

2 tablespoons of chives (finely chopped)

Spray olive oil

¼ cup of polenta

1 egg (lightly beaten)

¼ cup of whole meal self-rising flour

1 teaspoon of lemon juice

2 x 95g can salmon in Springwater (drained)

Directions:

1. First, you combine polenta and water in a medium-size bowl.
2. After which you allow to sit for 5 minutes.
3. After that, you stir through egg and milk.
4. At this point, fold in flour and mix until mixture is smooth.
5. This is when you heat a non-stick frying pan over medium-low heat.
6. Furthermore, spray with olive oil.
7. After which you pour 2-teaspoon portions of mixture around the pan, allowing room for spreading.
8. Then, cook for 1 minute or until bubbles appear.
9. In addition, turn and cook for a further 30 seconds or until golden brown; repeat with remaining mixture.
10. After that, combine cottage cheese, lemon juice and 1 tablespoon chives.

11. Finally, spread pikelets with cottage cheese mix and top with salmon and chives.

Bruschetta

Ingredients

4 Roma tomatoes (chopped)

1 clove garlic (peeled and finely chopped)

2 teaspoons of olive oil

Black pepper (to season)

4 slices Italian bread or sourdough

½ small red onion (peeled and chopped)

2 teaspoons of balsamic vinegar

2 tablespoons of torn basil leaves

Directions:

1. First, toast or chargrill bread.
2. After which you combine remaining ingredients in a small bowl.
3. After that, let stand for 10 minutes.
4. Then cut the bread slices in half and spoon over tomato mixture.

Cheesy salmon frittatas

Ingredients

- 5 tablespoons of reduced fat ricotta cheese

- 1 large zucchini (grated)

- 2 tablespoons parsley (finely chopped)

- 8 eggs

- 3 tablespoons of whole meal plain flour

- 1 x 95g can salmon in Springwater (drained)

- ¾ cup (about 115g) frozen peas (thawed)

Directions:

1. Meanwhile, heat oven to 160°C.
2. After which you grease with spray oil and line the bases of 4 holes of a large, muffin tin or mini loaf pan with rounds of baking paper.
3. After that, whisk the eggs and ricotta together in a medium bowl.
4. Then, stir through grated zucchini, flour, salmon, peas and parsley.
5. Furthermore, ladle mixture into prepared muffin tins.
6. Finally, bake for 20-25 minutes or until filling is set and golden.

Tip: remember, the frittatas will keep in an airtight container in the fridge for up to 4 days.

Energy balls

Ingredients

½ cup plain, unsalted almonds (dry roasted and chopped)

¼ cup plain (unsalted cashews)

¼ cup of sesame seeds

½ cup of dried figs (chopped)

½ cup of brown puffed rice

¼ cup of maple syrup

¼ cup of tahini

Directions:

1. First, you combine figs and almonds in a food processor for approximately 1 minute or until mixture forms a medium-fine consistency.
2. After which you add puffed rice and cashews and pulse for an additional 15 seconds.
3. After that, pour maple syrup and tahini into mixture while the motor is still running, until mixture reaches a moist consistency that sticks slightly between two fingers.
4. Then use damp hands roll a heaped teaspoon into a ball and coat with sesame seeds.
5. At this point, repeat to make 12 balls.
6. Finally, store in airtight container in the pantry for up to 3 weeks until ready to eat.

Tips:

If you want to dry roast almonds, I suggest you preheat oven to 180°C, place almonds on a cooking tray and bake for 8-10 minutes.

Healthy nachos

Ingredients

Spray olive oil

1 small red onion (finely chopped)

2 carrots (peeled, grated)

400g can no added salt diced tomato

100g can no added salt corn kernels (drained, rinsed)

Coriander sprigs (to serve)

2 small whole meal tortillas (cut into triangles)

1 garlic clove (crushed)

½ red capsicum (seeded, finely chopped)

1 teaspoon of Mexican chili powder

200g can no added salt red kidney beans (drained, rinsed)

¼ cup (about 30g) grated reduced fat mozzarella

Directions:

1. Meanwhile, heat the oven to 180°C.
2. After which you spray a deep medium sized rectangle baking tray with olive oil.
3. After that, prepare another large baking tray with baking paper.
4. Then, spread the pita triangles out in a single layer on the baking tray.
5. At this point, spray with olive oil and bake for about 5 minutes or until golden in the preheated oven.
6. In the meantime, spray a medium-size saucepan over medium heat.

7. This is when you add onion and garlic; cook, stirring, for 2 to 3 minutes or until soft.
8. Furthermore, add carrot, capsicum, and chili powder.
9. After which you cook, stirring occasionally, for 2 to 3 minutes or until capsicum is just tender.
10. In addition, add beans, diced tomatoes, and corn; bring to the boil.
11. After that, reduce heat to low and simmer for 4-5 minutes or until the mixture has slightly thickened; set aside.
12. Then place baked pita chips into a deep baking tray and top with tomato, bean and corn mix plus grated cheese.
13. Finally, bake for 10 minutes, until bubbling and golden.
14. You can top with coriander sprigs to serve.

Grilled stone fruit with crushed pecans and a maple glaze

Ingredients

olive oil spray

½ cup pecans (chopped)

4 medium stone fruits (e.g. yellow peaches, nectarines), halved and stones removed

4 teaspoons of maple syrup

400g reduced fat vanilla Greek yoghurt

Directions:

1. First, heat a char-grill over medium to low heat and spray generously with olive oil to prevent the stone fruits sticking.
2. After which you brush each fruit half with ½ teaspoon maple syrup.
3. After that, place cut-side down of the peach and grill for 8-10 minutes, or until grill marks appear and peaches are caramelized.
4. Then you divide the Greek yoghurt amongst the bowls and top with the grilled fruit and chopped pecans.

Mini berry and yoghurt pavlova

Ingredients

1 cup of caster sugar

400g reduced fat Greek yoghurt

300g blueberries

150ml egg whites (approximately 4 eggs)

1 teaspoon of white vinegar

300g strawberries (diced)

Directions:

1. Meanwhile, heat oven to 150°C.
2. After which you line a large baking tray with non-stick baking paper.
3. After that, place the egg whites in the bowl of an electric mixer and whisk on high speed until stiff peaks form.
4. Then you gradually add the sugar, 1 tablespoon at a time, waiting 30 seconds between each tablespoon.
5. At this point, whisk for 6 minutes or until stiff and glossy.
6. Furthermore, scrape the sides of the electric mixer, add the vinegar and whisk for 2 minutes or until glossy and combined.
7. This is when you spoon 6 rounds onto the baking tray.
8. After which you reduce the oven temperature to 120°C and bake for 30 minutes or until crisp to touch.
9. In addition, cool in the oven for 1 hour.
10. Finally, top meringues with yoghurt and fresh berries.

Oat based fruit crumble

Ingredients

Crumble:

¾ cup of rolled oats

1 tablespoon of olive oil

¼ cup of whole meal plain flour

1 teaspoon of cinnamon

2 tablespoons of pure maple syrup

Filling:

1 teaspoon of ground cinnamon

2 tablespoons of water

3 Granny Smith apples (cored and peeled, thinly sliced)

½ teaspoon of ground nutmeg

Directions:

Meanwhile, heat oven to 200°C.

After which you combine flour, cinnamon, rolled oats, maple syrup and olive oil into a bowl and mix until combined.

To prepare the filling:

1. First, combine cinnamon, apples and nutmeg in a large bowl and stir until well combined.
2. After that, transfer to a 1.5-liter ovenproof dish and add water.
3. Then, spoon crumble mixture over the apples.

4. Finally, you bake for 35-40 minutes, or until golden and apples are soft.

Made in the USA
Columbia, SC
14 January 2021